37 Heart Disease Juice Recipe Remedies:

Begin to Feel the Difference with These Easy to Prepare Juice Recipes!

By

Joe Correa CSN

COPYRIGHT

© 2017 Live Stronger Faster Inc.

All rights reserved

Reproduction or translation of any part of this work beyond that permitted by section 107 or 108 of the 1976 United States Copyright Act without the permission of the copyright owner is unlawful.

This publication is designed to provide accurate and authoritative information in regard to the subject matter covered. It is sold with the understanding that neither the author nor the publisher is engaged in rendering medical advice. If medical advice or assistance is needed, consult with a doctor. This book is considered a guide and should not be used in any way detrimental to your health. Consult with a physician before starting this nutritional plan to make sure it's right for you.

ACKNOWLEDGEMENTS

This book is dedicated to my friends and family that have had mild or serious illnesses so that you may find a solution and make the necessary changes in your life.

37 Heart Disease Juice Recipe Remedies:

Begin to Feel the Difference with These Easy to Prepare Juice Recipes!

By

Joe Correa CSN

CONTENTS

Copyright

Acknowledgements

About The Author

Introduction

37 Heart Disease Juice Recipe Remedies: Begin to Feel the Difference with These Easy to Prepare Juice Recipes!

Additional Titles from This Author

ABOUT THE AUTHOR

After years of Research, I honestly believe in the positive effects that proper nutrition can have over the body and mind. My knowledge and experience has helped me live healthier throughout the years and which I have shared with family and friends. The more you know about eating and drinking healthier, the sooner you will want to change your life and eating habits.

Nutrition is a key part in the process of being healthy and living longer so get started today. The first step is the most important and the most significant.

INTRODUCTION

37 Heart Disease Juice Recipe Remedies: Begin to Feel the Difference with These Easy to Prepare Juice Recipes!

By Joe Correa CSN

Many people believe that heart disease is a problem that only happens to other people. Furthermore, people believe that they are too young or too healthy to have any problems with their heart. This, unfortunately, is not true.

Heart disease is the number one cause of death in the world, for both men and women. A wide range of conditions that affect the heart can become a serious problem for middle-aged as well as older people. Once the disease is diagnosed, it lasts for life which is why your doctor will advise some medications and lifestyle changes. This part is crucial in keeping the condition under control. On the contrary, heart disease will get worse over time.

Fortunately, changing lifestyle choices, a healthy diet, and moderate exercise can reduce the risk of getting heart disease, or atleast, control the existing condition. But first, you have to understand that there are two major risk factors that lead to heart disease.

1. **Family history** is a huge risk factor when considering heart disease that can't be controlled. If this is your case, then a proper physical exam should be scheduled promptly.
2. **Unhealthy lifestyle choices** like smoking, obesity, physical inactivity, alcoholism, stress, increased cholesterol levels and diabetes are among the main causes of heart disease. Fortunately, these outside factors can easily be controlled with a proper diet and a healthy lifestyle.

Having just one of these risk factors is a serious condition and extremely dangerous and should be prevented and treated as soon as possible.

This collection of delicious and tasty juice recipes will help you clean your body and improve your health. These juices are based on a variety of fresh fruits and vegetables that are proven to help clean blood vessels and ease the everyday functions of your heart. Preventing heart disease has never been easier, it only takes a couple of minutes in the morning to prepare your favorite, heart-friendly juice recipe which will reduce your cholesterol levels, clean your entire digestive tract, and keep your blood vessels in check.

I hope this book will be your first step in making some positive changes in your life. Enjoy these recipes and have a wonderful life!

37 HEART DISEASE JUICE RECIPE REMEDIES: BEGIN TO FEEL THE DIFFERENCE WITH THESE EASY TO PREPARE JUICE RECIPES!

1. **Watermelon Grapefruit Juice**

Ingredients:

2 cups of watermelon, seeded

1 large grapefruit, chopped

2 cups of blueberries

1 tbsp of liquid honey

2 oz of water

Preparation:

Cut the watermelon lengthwise. For 2 cups, you will need about 2 large wedges. Peel and cut into chunks. Remove the seeds and set aside. Reserve the rest of the melon for some other juices.

Peel the grapefruit and divide into wedges. Set aside.

Wash the blueberries under cold running water. Drain and set aside.

Now, process blueberries, watermelon, and grapefruit in a juicer. Transfer to serving glasses and stir in the honey and water.

Refrigerate for 15 minutes before serving.

Enjoy!

Nutritional information per serving: Kcal: 375, Protein: 5.9g, Carbs: 92.1g, Fats: 1.7g

2. Carrot Apple Juice

Ingredients:

2 large carrots

1 large Honeycrisp apple, cored

2 large kiwis, peeled

1 cup of mint, chopped

1 large orange, peeled

2 oz of water

Preparation:

Wash the carrots and cut into thick slices. Set aside

Wash the apple and remove the core. Cut into bite-sized pieces and set aside.

Peel the kiwis and cut lengthwise in half. Set aside.

Wash the fresh mint and roughly chop it. Set aside.

Now, combine kiwis, carrots, apple, and mint in a juicer and process until juiced. Transfer to serving glasses and add some ice before serving.

Enjoy!

Nutritional information per serving: Kcal: 292, Protein: 6.1g, Carbs: 88.6g, Fats: 1.8g

3. Cabbage Lemon Juice

Ingredients:

1 cup of purple cabbage, torn

1 large lemon, peeled

2 cups of Brussels sprouts

2 cups of fennel

1 cup of beet greens, torn

1 large cucumber

Preparation:

Combine cabbage and beet greens in a colander and wash under cold running water. Torn with hands and set aside.

Wash the Brussels sprouts and trim off the outer leaves. Cut in half and set aside.

Wash the fennel bulb and trim off the wilted outer layers. Cut into small chunks and set aside.

Wash the cucumber and cut into thick slices. Set aside.

Now, combine Brussels sprouts, fennel, cabbage, beet greens, and cucumber in a juicer and process until juiced.

Transfer to serving glasses and add few ice cubes before serving.

Enjoy!

Nutritional information per serving: Kcal: 154, Protein: 12.8g, Carbs: 53g, Fats: 1.5g

4.　Zucchini Pomegranate Juice

Ingredients:

1 large zucchini, seeded

1 cup of pomegranate seeds

1 large orange, peeled

3 large kiwis, peeled

1 large lime, peeled

Preparation:

Wash the zucchini and cut in half. Scoop out the seeds using a spoon. Cut into small chunks and set aside.

Cut the top of the pomegranate fruit using a sharp knife. Slice down to each of the white membranes inside of the fruit. Pop the seeds into a measuring cup and set aside.

Peel the orange and divide into wedges. Set aside.

Peel the kiwis and cut lengthwise in half. Set aside.

Peel the lime and cut lengthwise in half. Set aside.

Now, process kiwis, zucchini, lime, pomegranate seeds, and orange in a juicer.

Transfer to a serving glasses and add some ice cubes before serving.

Nutritional information per serving: Kcal: 183, Protein: 8.5g, Carbs: 52.6g, Fats: 1.6g

5. Mango Banana Juice

Ingredients:

1 cup of mango, chunked

1 large banana, sliced

1 large carrot, sliced

1 whole lime, peeled

1 small Golden Delicious apple, cored

¼ tsp of cinnamon, ground

Preparation:

Peel the mango and cut into small chunks. Fill the measuring cup and reserve the rest in the refrigerator. Set aside.

Peel the banana and cut into slices. Set aside.

Wash and peel the carrot. Cut into thin slices and set aside.

Peel the lime and cut lengthwise in half. Set aside.

Wash the apple and cut in half. Remove the core and chop into bite-sized pieces. Set aside.

Now, combine carrot, lime, mango, banana, and apple in a juicer and process until juiced. Transfer to a serving glass and stir in the cinnamon.

Add some ice and serve immediately.

Nutrition information per serving: Kcal: 290, Protein: 4.1g, Carbs: 83.9g, Fats: 1.5g

6. Kale Asparagus Juice

Ingredients:

1 cup of kale, chopped

1 cup of asparagus, trimmed

1 large fennel bulb

1 large artichoke head

1 cup of Brussel sprouts, trimmed

1 cup of Swiss chard, chopped

¼ tsp of Cayenne pepper, ground

Preparation:

Combine kale and Swiss chard in a colander and wash under cold running water. Roughly chop it and set aside.

Wash the asparagus and trim off the woody ends. Cut into small pieces and set aside.

Wash the fennel bulb and trim off the wilted outer layers. Cut into small chunks and set aside.

Trim off the outer leaves of the artichoke. Wash it and cut into bite-sized pieces. Set aside.

Wash the Brussel sprouts and trim off the outer layers. Cut in half and set aside.

Now, process fennel, artichoke, kale, asparagus, Brussel sprouts, and Swiss chard in a juicer. Transfer to serving glasses and stir in the Cayenne pepper.

Refrigerate for 10 minutes before serving.

Nutritional information per serving: Kcal: 154, Protein: 17.6g, Carbs: 54.4g, Fats: 1.8g

7. Orange Mint Juice

Ingredients:

1 large orange

2 cups of fresh mint, torn

2 cups of fresh raspberries

1 large green apple, cored

1 large lime

2 oz of water

Preparation:

Peel the orange and divide into wedges. Set aside.

Wash the mint thoroughly and torn with hands. Set aside.

Wash the raspberries under cold running water and set aside.

Peel the apple and remove the core. Cut into bite-sized pieces and set aside.

Peel the lime and cut lengthwise in half. Set aside.

Now, process raspberries, mint, orange, apple, and lime in a juicer. Transfer to serving glasses and stir in the water.

Add some ice and serve immediately.

Nutritional information per serving: Kcal: 258, Protein: 7.6g, Carbs: 90.1g, Fats: 2.7g

8. Lemon Honey Juice

Ingredients:

1 large lemon, peeled

1 tbsp of liquid honey

1 cup of blueberries

1 large orange, peeled

1 large green apple, cored

Preparation:

Peel the lemon and cut lengthwise in half. Set aside.

Place the blueberries in a colander and wash under cold running water. Drain and set aside.

Peel the orange and divide into wedges. Set aside.

Wash the apple and remove the core. Cut into bite-sized pieces and set aside.

Now, combine blueberries, lemon, orange, and apple in a juicer and process until juiced.

Transfer to serving glasses and stir in the liquid honey.

Add few ice cubes or refrigerate before serving

Nutritional information per serving: Kcal: 305, Protein: 4.3g, Carbs: 76.5g, Fats: 1.3g

9.   Grapefruit Lime Juice

Ingredients:

2 large grapefruits

1 large lime

2 cups of celery, chopped

2 large carrots

1 ginger root slice, 1-inch

2 oz of water

Preparation:

Peel the grapefruits and divide into wedges. Set aside.

Peel the lime lengthwise in half. Set aside.

Wash the celery and chop into small pieces. About 2 large stalks will be enough. Set aside.

Wash the carrots and cut into thick slices. Set aside.

Peel the ginger slice and set aside.

Now, process celery, grapefruits, lime, carrots, and ginger in a juicer. Transfer to serving glasses and stir in the water.

Refrigerate for 15 minutes before serving.

Enjoy!

Nutritional information per serving: Kcal: 250, Protein: 6.7g, Carbs: 76.3g, Fats: 1.4g

10. Kiwi Celery Juice

Ingredients:

1 large kiwi, peeled

3 celery stalks

½ medium-sized grapefruit, peeled

1 large lemon, peeled

¼ tsp of ginger, ground

¼ tsp of Cayenne pepper, ground

A handful of watercress

Preparation:

Peel the kiwi and cut into halves. Set aside.

Wash the grapefruit and cut into halves. Chop one half into small cubes and reserve the other half for later. Set aside.

Peel the lemon and cut into quarters. Set aside.

Wash the watercress in and roughly chop it.

Now, process kiwi, grapefruit, lemon, and celery in a juicer until juiced.

Transfer to serving glasses and stir in the Cayenne pepper and ginger. You can add a pinch of Himalayan salt, but this is optional.

Serve immediately.

Nutritional information per serving: Kcal: 61, Protein: 2.1g, Carbs: 20.4g, Fats: 1.1g

11. Cinnamon Mango Juice

Ingredients:

1 cup of mango, chunked

1 large peach, pitted

1 medium-sized Granny Smith's apple, cored

1 whole lemon, peeled

¼ tsp of cinnamon, ground

Preparation:

Peel the mango and cut into small chunks. Fill the measuring cup and reserve the rest in the refrigerator. Set aside.

Wash the peach and cut in half. Remove the pit and chop into small pieces. Set aside.

Wash the apple and cut lengthwise in half. Remove the core and chop into bite-sized pieces. Set aside.

Peel the lemon and cut lengthwise in half. Set aside.

Now, combine peach, apple, lemon, and mango in a juicer and process until juiced. Transfer to a serving glass and stir in the cinnamon.

Add some crushed ice and serve immediately.

Enjoy!

Nutrition information per serving: Kcal: 236, Protein: 4.3g, Carbs: 69.5g, Fats: 1.5g

12. Apple Kale Juice

Ingredients:

1 large green apple, cored

1 cup of fresh kale

3 large kiwis

1 large lemon

1 cup of fresh mint

A handful of fresh spinach

3 oz of water

Preparation:

Wash the apple and remove the core. Cut into bite-sized pieces and set aside.

Wash kale, mint, and spinach and combine in a large bowl. Pour hot water enough to cover the ingredients. Let it soak for 10 minutes. Drain and torn with hands. Set aside.

Peel the kiwis and lemon. Cut lengthwise in half and set aside.

Now, process kiwis, lemon, kale, mint, spinach, and apple in a juicer. Transfer to serving glasses and stir in the water.

Add some ice and serve immediately.

Enjoy!

Nutritional information per serving: Kcal: 246, Protein: 8.6g, Carbs: 74.5g, Fats: 2.6g

13. Sweet Beet Juice

Ingredients:

1 cup of beets, trimmed and chopped

3 large carrots

1 large cucumber

1 large orange, peeled

2 oz of water

½ tsp of agave nectar

Preparation:

Wash the beets and trim off the green parts. Cut into bite-sized pieces and fill the measuring cup. Reserve the rest for some other juice.

Wash the carrots and cut into thick slices. Set aside.

Wash the cucumber and cut into thick slices. Set aside.

Peel the orange and divide into wedges. Set aside.

Now, combine carrots, beets, cucumber, and orange in a juicer and process until juiced.

Transfer to serving glasses and stir in the water and agave nectar. Add some ice and serve immediately.

Nutritional information per serving: Kcal: 296, Protein: 7.9g, Carbs: 86.2g, Fats: 1.3g

14. Cantaloupe Orange Juice

Ingredients:

2 cups of blackberries

1 cup of cantaloupe, diced

1 large orange

1 large lemon

1 small Granny Smith's apple

Preparation:

Cut the cantaloupe in half. Scoop out the seeds and flesh. Cut two wedges and peel them. Chop into chunks and set aside. Reserve the rest of the cantaloupe in a refrigerator.

Peel the orange and divide into wedges. Set aside.

Place the blackberries in a colander and wash under cold running water. Drain and set aside.

Peel the lemon and cut lengthwise in half. Set aside.

Wash the apple and remove the core. Cut into bite-sized pieces and set aside.

Now, combine blackberries, cantaloupe, orange, lemon, and apple in a juicer and process until juiced. Transfer to serving glasses and refrigerate for 10 minutes before serving.

Enjoy!

Nutritional information per serving: Kcal: 258, Protein: 8.3g, Carbs: 87g, Fats: 2.4g

15. Tomato Lemon Juice

Ingredients:

1 cup of cherry tomatoes, halved

1 large lemon, peeled

1 cup of basil, torn

1 large red bell pepper, seeded

1 rosemary sprig

¼ tsp of Himalayan salt

Preparation:

Wash the tomatoes and place in a bowl. Cut in half and reserve the juice while cutting. Set aside.

Peel the lemon and cut lengthwise in half. Set aside.

Wash the basil thoroughly under cold running water using a colander. Drain and torn with hands. Set aside.

Wash the bell pepper and cut in half. Remove the seeds and cut into small pieces. Set aside.

Now, combine tomatoes, basil, pepper, and lemon in a juicer and process until juiced. Transfer to serving glasses and stir in the salt. Sprinkle with some rosemary for some extra taste.

Refrigerate for 10 minutes before serving.

Nutritional information per serving: Kcal: 189, Protein: 19.5g, Carbs: 53.1g, Fats: 2.6g

16. Garlic Kale Juice

Ingredients:

4 fresh kale leaves

1 garlic clove, peeled

2 large oranges, peeled

½ cup of fresh broccoli, chopped

3 large carrots

4 collard green leaves

¼ tsp of Himalayan salt

2 oz of water

Preparation:

Combine collard greens and kale in a colander and wash under cold running water. Roughly chop and set aside.

Peel the garlic clove and set aside.

Peel the oranges and divide into wedges. Set aside.

Wash the broccoli and chop into small pieces. set aside.

Wash the carrots and cut into small pieces. set aside.

Process oranges, broccoli, carrots, collard greens, kale and garlic in a juicer. Transfer to serving glasses and stir in the Himalayan salt and water.

Serve immediately.

Nutritional information per serving: Kcal: 171, Protein: 9.2g, Carbs: 43.3g, Fats: 2.3g

17. Artichoke Zucchini Juice

Ingredients:

1 medium-sized artichoke, chopped

1 small zucchini, sliced

1 cup of sweet potatoes, cubed

1 whole lime, peeled

1 large carrot, sliced

¼ tsp of salt

¼ tsp of turmeric, ground

Preparation:

Wash the artichoke and trim off the outer leaves. Cut into small pieces and fill the measuring cup. Reserve the rest in the refrigerator.

Peel the zucchini and cut into thin slices. Set aside.

Peel the potatoes and cut into small cubes. Place in a deep pot and add 3 cups of water. Bring it to a boil and cook for 5 minutes. Remove from the heat and drain well. Set aside to cool completely.

Peel the lime and cut lengthwise in half. Set aside.

Wash and peel the carrot. Cut into thin slices and set aside.

Now, combine potatoes, artichoke, zucchini, lime, and carrots in a juicer and process until juiced. Transfer to a serving glass and stir in the salt and turmeric.

Refrigerate for 10 minutes before serving.

Nutrition information per serving: Kcal: 177, Protein: 8.6g, Carbs: 54.5g, Fats: 0.8g

18. Watermelon Kiwi Juice

Ingredients:

1 cup of watermelon

1 large kiwi

1 large orange

1 large green apple, cored

1 large guava

3 oz of coconut water

Preparation:

Cut the watermelon lengthwise. For one cup, you will need about one large wedge. Peel and cut into chunks. Remove the seeds and set aside. Reserve the rest of the melon for some other juices.

Peel the kiwi and cut lengthwise in half. Set aside.

Wash the guava and cut into chunks. If you are using large fruit, reserve the rest for some other recipe in a refrigerator.

Peel the orange and divide into wedges. Set aside.

Wash the apple and remove the core. Cut into bite-sized pieces and set aside.

Now, combine guava, watermelon, orange, kiwi, and apple in a juicer and process until juiced. Transfer to serving glasses and stir in the coconut water.

Add some ice or refrigerate before serving.

Enjoy!

Nutritional information per serving: Kcal: 264, Protein: 5.6g, Carbs: 73.8g, Fats: 1.6g

19. Cherry Vanilla Juice

Ingredients:

1 cup of cherries, pitted

1 cup of cranberries

3 whole apricots, pitted and chopped

1 small Golden Delicious apple, cored

1 tsp of vanilla extract

3 tbsp of coconut water

Preparation:

Rinse the cherries under cold running water. Drain and cut each cherry in half. Remove the pits and set aside.

Rinse the cranberries using a large colander. Drain and set aside.

Wash the apricots and cut in half. Remove the pits and chop into small pieces. Set aside.

Wash the apple and cut lengthwise in half. Remove the core and chop into small pieces. Set aside.

Now, combine cranberries, apricots, apple, and cherries in a juicer and process until juiced. Transfer to a serving glass and stir in the vanilla extract and coconut water.

Sprinkle with some finely chopped mint for some extra taste. However, it's optional.

Add few ice cubes and serve immediately.

Nutrition information per serving: Kcal: 216, Protein: 3.8g, Carbs: 66.1g, Fats: 1.1g

20. Apple Carrot Juice

Ingredients:

2 large apples, cored

2 large carrots

½ cup of fresh spinach

¼ tsp of ginger, ground

2 tbsp of fresh parsley

1 tbsp of flaxseeds

Preparation:

Wash the apples and remove the core. Cut into bite-sized pieces and set aside.

Wash and chop the carrots into small pieces. Set aside.

Wash the spinach thoroughly under cold running water. Drain and torn into small pieces. Set aside.

Now, process all in a juicer until well juiced. Transfer to serving glasses and stir in the ginger. Sprinkle with flaxseeds for some extra nutrients and serve immediately!

Nutritional information per serving: Kcal: 119, Protein: 4.3g, Carbs: 62.2g, Fats: 2.3g

21. Lemon Ginger Juice

Ingredients:

1 large lemon, peeled

½ tsp of ginger, ground

½ cup of cilantro

3 celery stalks

1 large green apple, cored

Preparation:

Peel the lemon and cut into quarters. Process in a juicer until juiced.

Wash the cilantro and chop it roughly. Set aside.

Wash the celery stalks and chop into small pieces. Set aside.

Wash the apple and remove the core. Cut into bite-sized pieces and set aside.

Now, process cilantro, celery, and apple. Transfer to serving glasses and stir in the ginger.

Refrigerate for 15 minutes or add some ice before serving.

Enjoy!

Nutritional information per serving: Kcal: 73, Protein: 2.2g, Carbs: 26.7g, Fats: 0.1g

22. Pumpkin Lettuce Juice

Ingredients:

1 cup of yellow pumpkin, chopped

1 cup of Romaine lettuce, chopped

2 large leeks, chopped

1 cup of asparagus, trimmed

2 tbsp of fresh parsley, chopped

1 large cucumber

Preparation:

Peel the pumpkin and cut in half. Scoop out the seeds using a spoon. Cut one large wedge and peel it. Cut into small chunks and fill the measuring cup. Reserve the rest for some other juice.

Combine lettuce and parsley in a colander and wash thoroughly under cold running water. Drain and roughly chop it.

Wash the leeks and chop into small pieces. Set aside.

Wash the asparagus and trim off the woody ends. Chop into small pieces and set aside.

Wash the cucumber and cut into thick slices. Set aside.

Now, process leeks, asparagus, pumpkin, lettuce, parsley, and cucumber in a juicer. Transfer to serving glasses and add some ice, or refrigerate for 20 minutes before serving.

Nutritional information per serving: Kcal: 185, Protein: 9.5g, Carbs: 50.8g, Fats: 1.3g

23. Broccoli Lemon Juice

Ingredients:

1 cup of fennel, chopped

1 cup of spinach, torn

1 cup of broccoli, chopped

1 whole lemon, peeled

1 whole lime, peeled

¼ tsp of ginger, ground

Preparation:

Wash the broccoli and trim off the outer leaves. Chop into small pieces and fill the measuring cup. Reserve the rest in the refrigerator.

Peel the lemon and lime. Cut lengthwise into halves. Set aside.

Trim off the fennel stalks and outer wilted layers. Wash and chop the fennel into bite-sized pieces. Fill the measuring cup and reserve the rest for later. Set aside.

Rinse the spinach thoroughly under cold running water and drain. Torn into small piecesand set aside.

Now, combine fennel, spinach, broccoli, lemon, and lime in a juicer. Process until juiced.

Transfer to a serving glass and stir in the ginger.

Add some crushed ice and serve immediately.

Nutrition information per serving: Kcal: 86, Protein: 10.5g, Carbs: 29.1g, Fats: 1.5g

24. Kale Artichoke Juice

Ingredients:

1 cup of kale, chopped

1 medium-sized artichoke head

3 cups of beet greens

1 bunch of spinach

1 large cucumber

3 tbsp of parsley, chopped

¼ tsp of Himalayan salt

Preparation:

Combine beet greens, spinach, kale and parsley in a large colander. Wash thoroughly under cold running water. Drain and roughly chop it. Set aside.

Trim off the outer wilted layers of the artichoke. Wash and cut into small pieces. Set aside.

Wash the cucumber and cut into thick slices. Set aside.

Now, combine beet greens, spinach, kale, artichoke, cucumber, and parsley in a juicer and process until juiced.

Transfer to serving glasses and stir in the salt.

Add some ice and serve immediately.

Nutritional information per serving: Kcal: 151, Protein: 21.6g, Carbs: 48.2g, Fats: 2.7g

25. Apple Cinnamon Juice

Ingredients:

1 small Golden Delicious apple, chopped

1 medium-sized orange, peeled

1 medium-sized pear, chopped

1 cup of beets, chopped

¼ tsp of cinnamon, ground

¼ tsp of ginger, ground

Preparation:

Wash the apple and cut lengthwise in half. Remove the core and cut into bite-sized pieces. Set aside.

Peel the orange and divide into wedges. Cut each wedge in half and set aside.

Wash the pear and cut in half. Remove the core and chop into small pieces. Set aside.

Wash the beets and trim off the green ends. Cut into slices and fill the measuring cup. Reserve the rest for later.

Now, combine orange, pear, beets, and apple in a juicer and process until juiced.

Transfer to a serving glass and stir in the cinnamon and ginger. Add some ice before serving.

Enjoy!

Nutrition information per serving: Kcal: 234, Protein: 4.4g, Carbs: 73.1g, Fats: 0.8g

26. Pumpkin Carrot Juice

Ingredients:

1 cup of pumpkin chunks

1 large carrot

1 large yellow apple, cored

1 large orange

¼ tsp of cinnamon, ground

3 oz of water

Preparation:

Peel the pumpkin and cut in half. Scoop out the seeds using a spoon. Cut one large wedge and peel it. Cut into small chunks and set aside. Reserve the rest for later.

Wash the carrot and cut into thick slices. Set aside.

Wash the apple and remove the core. Cut into bite-sized pieces and set aside.

Peel the orange and divide into wedges. Set aside.

Now, process pumpkin, apple, carrot, and orange in a juicer. Transfer to serving glasses and stir in the cinnamon and water.

Add few ice cubes and serve immediately.

Enjoy!

Nutritional information per serving: Kcal: 220, Protein: 4.1g, Carbs: 65.3g, Fats: 0.8g

27. Cantaloupe Pineapple Juice

Ingredients:

1 cup of cantaloupe, peeled

½ pineapple, peeled

2 large green apples, cored

½ cup of fresh kale

Preparation:

Peel and chop the cantaloupe into small cubes. Remove the seeds and set aside.

Peel the pineapple and cut into small chunks. Set aside.

Wash the apples and remove the core. Cut into bite-sized pieces and set aside.

Wash thoroughly the kale and soak in water for 10 minutes. Set aside.

Process cantaloupe, apple, pineapple, and kale in a juicer until nicely juiced. Transfer to serving glasses and add some ice before serving.

You can add some liquid honey to taste, but this is optional.

Enjoy!

Nutritional information per serving: Kcal: 115, Protein: 1.2g, Carbs: 28.8g, Fats: 1.2g

28. Lime Watercress Juice

Ingredients:

3 large limes, peeled

1 cup of watercress

1 cup of beets, trimmed

1 large green apple, cored

1 large cucumber

Preparation:

Peel the limes and cut lengthwise in half. Set aside.

Wash the watercress thoroughly under cold running water. Drain and set aside.

Wash the beets and trim off the green ends. Cut into bite-sized pieces and set aside.

Wash the apple and remove the core. Cut into bite-sized pieces. Set aside.

Wash the cucumber and cut into thick slices. Set aside.

Now, combine beets, limes, watercress, apple, and cucumber in a juicer and process until juiced.

Add some ice and serve.

Nutritional information per serving: Kcal: 211, Protein: 6.4g, Carbs: 63.5g, Fats: 1.1g

29. Kiwi Apple Juice

Ingredients:

2 large kiwis, peeled

1 large Fuji apple, cored

2 cups of blueberries

1 cup of watermelon, seeded

2 oz of coconut water

Preparation:

Peel the kiwis and cut lengthwise in half. Set aside.

Wash the apple and remove the core. Cut into bite-sized pieces and set aside.

Wash the blueberries under cold running water using a colander. Drain and set aside.

Cut the watermelon in half. Cut one large wedge and peel it. Chop into small chunks and remove the seeds. Fill the measuring cup and refrigerate the rest for some other juice.

Now, combine blueberries, kiwis, apple, and watermelon in a juicer and process until juiced. Transfer to serving glasses and stir in coconut water.

Add some ice and serve immediately.

Nutritional information per serving: Kcal: 315, Protein: 7.2g, Carbs: 97.9g, Fats: 2.8g

30. Beet Celery Juice

Ingredients:

1 cup of beets, sliced

1 cup of celery, cut into bite-sized pieces

1 cup of avocado, cubed

1 whole lemon, peeled

1 oz of water

Preparation:

Wash the beets and trim off the green ends. Slightly peel and cut into thin slices. Fill the measuring cup and reserve the rest for later.

Wash the celery and cut into bite-sized pieces. Fill the measuring cup and reserve the rest in the refrigerator.

Peel the avocado and cut lengthwise in half. Remove the pit and cut into small cubes. Fill the measuring cup and reserve the rest in the refrigerator. Set aside.

Peel the lemon and cut lengthwise in half. Set aside.

Now, combine avocado, beets, celery, and lemon in a juicer. Process until juiced.

Transfer to a serving glass and stir in the water. Refrigerate for 10 minutes before serving.

Nutrition information per serving: Kcal: 264, Protein: 6.5g, Carbs: 34.2g, Fats: 22.5g

31. Cherry Mint Juice

Ingredients:

1 cup of cherries, pitted

2 tbsp of fresh mint, chopped

2 cups of green grapes

1 medium-sized Fuji apple, cored

1 tbsp of liquid honey

2 oz of water

Preparation:

Combine grapes and cherries in a large colander. Wash under cold running water and drain. Cut the cherries in half and remove the pits. Set aside.

Wash the mint and roughly chop it. Set aside.

Wash the apple and remove the core. Cut into bite-sized pieces and set aside.

Now, combine grapes, cherries, apple, and mint in a juicer and process until juiced.

Transfer to serving glasses and add some ice before serving.

Nutritional information per serving: Kcal: 369, Protein: 3.5g, Carbs: 104g, Fats: 1.4g

32. Grapefruit Kale Juice

Ingredients:

½ cup of grapefruit, chopped

3-4 fresh kale leaves

2 large oranges, peeled

1 tsp of liquid honey

¼ tsp of ginger, ground

Preparation:

Wash the grapefruit and cut into halves. Cut one-half into small pieces. Reserve the other half in a fridge.

Wash the kale leaves and roughly chop it.

Peel the oranges and divide into wedges. Set aside.

Now, process oranges, grapefruit, and kale in a juicer. Transfer to serving glasses and add some water to adjust the thickness if needed.

Stir in the liquid honey and ginger. Add some ice and serve immediately.

Nutritional information per serving: Kcal: 128, Protein: 7.3g, Carbs: 34.5g, Fats: 1.1g

33. Cucumber Apple Juice

Ingredients:

1 cup of cucumber, sliced

1 medium-sized Golden Delicious apple, cored

1 large banana, peeled

2 whole kiwis, peeled

1 cup of fresh mint, torn

Preparation:

Wash the cucumber and cut into thin slices. Fill the measuring cup and reserve the rest for later. Set aside.

Wash the apple and cut lengthwise in half. Remove the core and cut into bite-sized pieces. Set aside.

Peel the banana and cut into thin slices. Set aside.

Peel the kiwis and cut lengthwise in half. Set aside.

Rinse the mint thoroughly under cold running water and drain. Torn into small pieces and set aside.

Now, combine kiwis, cucumber, apple, and banana in a juicer and process until juiced. Transfer to a serving glass and add some ice.

Serve immediately.

Nutrition information per serving: Kcal: 272, Protein: 4.8g, Carbs: 79.8g, Fats: 1.7g

34. Pepper Shallot Juice

Ingredients:

1 large bell pepper, seeded

1 small shallot

2 large tomatoes, halved

2 garlic cloves, peeled

3 large cucumbers

1 large lime, peeled

¼ cup of fresh cilantro

Preparation:

Wash the bell pepper and cut into halves. Remove the seeds and chop into small pieces.

Wash the shallots and chop into small pieces set aside.

Wash the tomatoes and place them in a medium bowl. Cut into quarters or small pieces. Reserve the juice while cutting and pour it into serving glasses.

Wash the cucumbers and chop into small pieces. Set aside.

Peel the lime and cut into quarters. Set aside.

Wash the cilantro and roughly chop it. Set aside.

Peel the garlic cloves and set aside.

Process the tomatoes, cucumbers, bell pepper, shallots, lime, garlic, and cilantro. Transfer to serving glasses and refrigerate for 20 minutes before serving.

Nutritional information per serving: Kcal: 109, Protein: 6.4g, Carbs: 38.5g, Fats: 1.2g

35. Fennel Orange Juice

Ingredients:

1 small fennel

1 large orange, peeled

6 medium-sized radishes

5 large celery stalks

1 large cucumber

Preparation:

Trim off the fennel stalks and wilted outer layers. Wash and cut into bite-sized pieces and set aside.

Peel the orange and divide into wedges.

Wash and cut the radishes into small pieces. Set aside.

Wash the celery and roughly chop into pieces. set aside.

Wash the cucumber and chop into small pieces.

Process all in a juicer, one at a time. Transfer to serving glasses and add some water to adjust the thickness, if needed.

Add some ice and serve.

Enjoy!

Nutritional information per serving: Kcal: 110, Protein: 6.1g, Carbs: 28.7g, Fats: 1.2g

36. Celery Apple Juice

Ingredients:

4 celery stalks

1 large green apple, cored

½ cup of green cabbage

3 large carrots

1 large lemon, peeled

1 tbsp of liquid honey

Preparation:

Wash the celery stalks and cut into small chunks. Set aside.

Wash the cabbage and roughly chop it. Set aside.

Peel the lemon and cut into quarters. Set aside.

Wash carrots and celery. Cut into small pieces and place in a medium bowl.

Wash the apple and remove the core. Cut into bite-sized pieces and set aside.

Now, first process the cabbage, then celery, apple, carrots, and lemon. Transfer to serving glasses and stir in the liquid honey.

Add water to adjust the thickness of the juice if you like. However, this is optional.

Refrigerate for about 5 minutes before serving.

Nutritional information per serving: Kcal: 162, Protein: 3.1g, Carbs: 39.3g, Fats: 0.1g

37. Plum Lime Juice

Ingredients:

1 whole plum, pitted and chopped

1 whole lime, peeled

1 medium-sized Red Delicious apple, cored

1 cup of raspberries

1 oz of water

Preparation:

Wash the plum and cut in half. Remove the pit and chop into small pieces. Set aside.

Peel the lime and cut lengthwise in half. Cut into quarters and set aside.

Place the raspberries in a colander and rinse well under cold running water. Drain and fill the measuring cup. Reserve the rest in the refrigerator. Set aside.

Wash the apple and cut lengthwise in half. Remove the core and cut into bite-sized pieces. Set aside.

Now, combine raspberries, lime, apple, and plum in a juicer and process until juiced. Transfer to a serving glass and stir in the water.

Refrigerate for 10 minutes before serving.

Nutrition information per serving: Kcal: 173, Protein: 2.7g, Carbs: 55.7g, Fats: 1.4g

ADDITIONAL TITLES FROM THIS AUTHOR

70 Effective Meal Recipes to Prevent and Solve Being Overweight: Burn Fat Fast by Using Proper Dieting and Smart Nutrition

By Joe Correa CSN

48 Acne Solving Meal Recipes: The Fast and Natural Path to Fixing Your Acne Problems in Less Than 10 Days!

By Joe Correa CSN

41 Alzheimer's Preventing Meal Recipes: Reduce or Eliminate Your Alzheimer's Condition in 30 Days or Less!

By Joe Correa CSN

70 Effective Breast Cancer Meal Recipes: Prevent and Fight Breast Cancer with Smart Nutrition and Powerful Foods

By Joe Correa CSN

www.ingramcontent.com/pod-product-compliance
Lightning Source LLC
Chambersburg PA
CBHW030301030426
42336CB00009B/480